Hospitals : their Origin and Evolution

John Foote

Hospitals : their Origin and Evolution

LM Publishers

"Originally, *hospital* meant a place where strangers or visitors were received; in the course of time, its use was restricted to institutions for the care of the sick. This modification is incidental to the long development through which the hospital itself has passed under the varying influences of religious, political, and economic conditions, and of social and scientific progress. Viewed in a large way the typical modern hospital represents natural human solicitude for suffering, ennobled by Christian charity and made efficient by the abundant resources of medical skill..."

- *James J. Walsh*

The story of the birth and evolution of the hospital is a record of the conquest of barbarism by civilization and of the triumph of Christian altruism over the selfishness of the pagan ideal. Bargaining, trading, warring, the nations of the earth have struggled upward along the difficult highway of achievement, making slow but certain progress in the betterment of humanity. Always this approach toward the ideal has been characterized by an increased interest in the welfare of the public as opposed to the individual, and exemplified in unselfish efforts to befriend the sick and friendless.

No better index, therefore, of the progress of any nation in ethics and altruism can be obtained than a report of its work in the building and management of hospitals.

In its origin the word *hospital* comes from early Christian days when it was used to designate a place where strangers and visitors were received and cared for. Whether or not hospitals proper existed in pre-Christian time is a much-debated question. The fact has been established that the Egyptians studied medicine and that the sick were brought to their temples to be healed by the priests. To some extent this practise was observed by the Greeks and by the Romans in their temples of Æsculapius.

There is certain evidence of the existence in pagan Rome of *Valetadinaria,* or dispensaries, for sick soldiers and slaves; but of the existence of hospitals proper, houses of refuge for the poor and the ill, we have no proof. Something more than mere civilization was necessary for the establishment of these tokens of man's regard for his fellow man.

In India, a country whose ancient moral code was less pagan, if not more Christian, than that of either Greece or Rome, hospitals for men and animals are described by two early Chinese explorers. Prescott states that hospitals existed in Mexico before the Conquest, but his documentary proof is indefinite. Gaelic literature is rich in traditions concerning the House of Sorrow, a hospital for the wounded of the Red Branch Knights who lived about 300 B.C. at Tara, the palace of the kings of the heroic age of Ireland. But on sifting the evidence, we are justified in assuming that the claim of the pre-Christian hospital rests largely on tradition, while proof is abundant that these institutions were liberally encouraged by the Christian Church.

There are many allusions in the New Testament concerning the healing of the sick, and Christ himself commanded his disciples to care for the ill and indigent. The practise of hospitality was enjoined as a virtue upon the early Christians; bishops, presbyters and deacons were especially obliged to practise this virtue and references to it are found in the Acts and most of the early commentaries. These documents tell us that in the bishop's house was a room set apart for the use of poor and ill travelers, designated as the hospitalium, or rest room. Harnack states that the bishop was also required to act as a physician. In this hospital inn, therefore, in name as well as in function, we find the legitimate, though remote, ancestor of the modern hospital.

The many epidemics occurring in the Soman empire, as the epidemic of Carthage in a.d. 252, described by St. Cyprian, 2 gave those who would care for the sick abundant employment. Many a wealthier Christian imitated the bishop's good example and established a hospitalium in his own house. But, hunted and persecuted as the sect was, there could be no organization of this work; their efforts must remain desultory and scattered until the ban was removed. So it is that the advent of the public hospital comes after the reign of Constantine, when a great increase in the number of Christians and the spread of poverty had made adequate individual effort by the bishops difficult if not impossible.

More than one writer has asserted that hospitals originated from three supposedly antagonistic influences, religion, war and science. This statement is not true for several reasons, but chiefly because history is opposed to it. There was plenty of fighting in pre-Christian days, but hospitals did not result from it. The Greeks had far more scientific knowledge than the Goths, yet the former did not build hospitals, while the latter did. Indeed, the real situation is outlined if we say that in the social ebullition produced among the nations of Europe by the introduction of Christianity, hospitals were the distillate and war and science the by-products.

The Christianity of the Lombards, the Goths and the Franks was a militant one. Scarcely had Clovis, the Prankish king, renounced his old gods than he commenced a holy war upon his unorthodox neighbors with the twofold object of converting them and obtaining dominion over their lands. In the dream of empire of the first great Charles the sword and the cross were close companions. Yet these early Frankish monarchs in the intervals between their wars were earnest in the building of hospitals. Long indeed after the hospital made its appearance came the university — so long, in fact, that the statement that the origin of the hospital owed much, if anything, to science is disproved chronologically. And this, too, without in the least minimizing the influence of the great medieval schools, such as Salerno and Montpellier, upon the hospitals of the middle ages.

But now to consider in brief detail the hospitals of early Christian era. We must first give our attention to the east, where the conversion of Constantine gave an impetus to the spread of Christian religion. Ratsinger asserts that a hospital was established at Constantinople by St. Zoticus during the reign of the first Christian emperor, but his authority for this statement is mythical. We have, however, documentary proof in the writings of St. Gregory, of Nazianus — whose brother ; by the way, was a physician — of the establishment of a hospital by St. Basil at Csesarea, in Cappadocia (a.d. 369).

According to Gregory, it was a veritable city with streets separating pavilions for various diseases and also workshops, industrial schools, convalescent homes and residences for attendants, nurses and physicians.

Indeed, the plan seems not unlike our most modern pavilion system; the ancient writer waxes enthusiastic in his praise of it, declaring it to be " a heaven upon earth."

Alexandria boasted a hospital in 610, founded by St. John the Almsgiver, and at about this same time Bishop Brassianus established one at Ephesus. Contemporaneous was the foundation in Constantinople of three hospitals, one by St. John Chrysostom, one by St. Pulcheria, sister of the Emperor Theodosius II., and one by St. Sampson. Thirty-five hospitals were erected in this one eastern city alone before the tenth century, according to the Constantinopolis Christiana of Du Cange. An orphanotrophium was established in the tenth century by Alexis I., and the Hospital of the Forty Martyrs by Isum II in the eleventh century. Such was the influence of these Eastern institutions that we find their Greek terminology influencing the names of early institutions of the west. In all the writings of later days concerning hospitals a house for sick people is called a "noscomium," for foundlings a "orphanotrophium," etc. Perhaps one of the best proofs we have of the activity of the Christians in hospital building is the fact that the Emperor Julian, called the Apostate, decreed that hospitals should be built to offset the influence of similar institutions which the Christians had inaugurated.

St. Jerome tells us of the hospital builded by Fabiola in Rome during the fifth century. Fabiola, a wealthy Roman lady, is probably our first Christian philanthropist. Pope Symmachus (495-514) built three hospitals in Rome during his pontificate, and these were maintained and additional ones built by his successors. But Stephen II surpassed his predecessors in the eighth century by restoring four ancient institutions and building three new ones.

The Arabs, speedily changing from a barbaric army to a cultivated and civilized people through their contact with Greek thought in the countries conquered by them, were not long in proving their enlightenment by the standard of hospital building. The first Arabian hospital was built at Damascus a.d. 707 by the Caliph el Welid. Virtually the real rise of Arabian science came with the accession to power of the Abbasides (a.d. 750). The Arab by this time was a mixed nation, in which the Persian element seemed to predominate. Hospitals under medical supervision were not uncommon, although infirmaries predominated. Nuburger states that infirmaries existed in no less than fourteen cities, including Bagdad, Antioch, Jericho, Medina, Mecca — in short, throughout the entire empire. The part played by pilgrimages to places of devotion among Christian nations in the evolution of the hospital was perhaps even more pronounced among the followers of Mohammed. Clinical teaching was done in several of the large hospitals of Damascus, special attention being given to medicine and diseases of the eye. The hospital, mosque and orphanage founded by al Munsur in the thirteenth century was one of the most notable Arabian charitable institutions and is said to have had a staff of forty-two physicians.

Probably the earliest hospital in France was the "Xenodochium" for pilgrims, established by King Childebert in the sixth century. The practise of making pilgrimages to the shrines and holy places was a custom of the pious coming more and more into vogue, and the monarch's action was a much-needed charity to the sick and weary travelers. The Council of Orleans (549) gave this establishment hearty approval.

Many hospitals arose in France during this and the succeeding century. For at just this period the Franklish empire, more than any other European country, was slowly tending toward the conditions which made it eventually a nation of city dwellers, dimly foreshadowing what came later with the establishment of industries, the foundation of guilds and the influence of trade and commerce on national life. At Autin, at Athis, at Paris, Aries and Eheims, we have records of the establishment of hospitals by kings, nobles and churchmen. The oldest hospital in the world still enduring, the famous Hotel Dieu, is attributed to Landry, Bishop of Paris, and its origin has been variously placed between a.d. 660 and 800. Lallemand's "Histoire de la Charite" finds the first extant written mention of it in a document of 829. This began as a cathedral hospital, and was one of a group of institutions growing up about the old churches, which, developing into small communities, formed the nucleus of many of the larger cities of the feudal period. Undoubtedly of much earlier origin was the Hospital Scothorum, which was built on the continent at a remote period by missionary Irish monks. This was destroyed and later was restored by order of the Council of Meux (a.d. 845). These were probably the same monks who founded the monasteries of Bobbio and St. Gall, and carried the art of illuminating manuscripts as well as the gospel itself to the semi-barbarous peoples beyond the Alps.

The idea of medical missionary work is not a new, but a very old, idea. Barbarous Europe was converted by medical missionaries ; practically all of the monasteries of the monks of the west did hospital work.

This monastic influence reached its zenith in the tenth century, and the most famous hospital-monastery of that day was the Benedictine abbey of Cluny, founded in 910, and commanding not only a local reputation, but famed through Italy and France.

Originally each monastery had its infirmary for inmates, and this under the laws of hospitality was open to sick travelers. Before long the crying need of medical aid extended the ministrations of the infirmary to the people of the neighborhood, or to any who might seek it. The monastery was the repository of medical as well as all other written knowledge of that period, and it has been proved that among the profane authors copied by the monks in their scriptoria were some of the classical authors on medicine.

We must not imagine that the cathedral hospital languished during the preponderance of monastic medicine; according to Virchow, 155 hospitals were founded in Germany alone from 1207 to 1577. With the growing importance of the hospital it is no surprise to find religious communities springing up whose chief and surpassing occupation was to be the care of the sick. The first of these was organized in Siena, a cradle of Italian genius, during the ninth century. Soror, the founder of the hospital of Santa Maria de la Scala, drew up the rules for its administration with his own hands. The management was largely in the hands of citizens, subject to the bishop's control. Many such communities were established in Italy and lived under the rule of St. Augustine.

From this time onward the religious orders strongly influenced hospital development. In the twelfth century the Beguines and Beghards were hospital orders which flourished especially throughout Belgium, France and Germany, while the Alexians and Antonines established and managed hospitals in various parts of Italy as well. Leprosy following in the wake of the crusades, special communities were formed to care for lepers. Thousands of leper houses arose in all parts of Europe — it is estimated that 2,000 existed in Germany alone.

The plague was eventually stamped out, an achievement in a public health campaign which would do credit to a much more enlightened age. Special communities also isolated and nursed cases of erysipelas known as St. Anthony's fire, St. Francis's fire, etc. But the most important event in the history of hospitals in the period we must now consider, the middle ages, was the foundation of the order of the Holy Ghost, resulting, as it did, in a golden age of hospital building extending from the thirteenth to the fifteenth century and not equalcd again till the hospital renaissance of the nineteenth century.

In the middle of the twelfth century Guy of Montpellier established the Hospital of the Holy Ghost in the city of his name. Montpellier was at that time the medical mecca of Europe and attracted students from remote cities. Not only the reputation of the hospital, but the order itself spread rapidly through France, building and managing hospitals.

Innocent III., the great militant pope, who did so much to strengthen the temporal power of the pontiff, had recently builded a hospital in Rome. It was characteristic of his genius that he foresaw the need of hospitals and the great work they might accomplish. He determined to promote their building not only in Rome and the Papal states, but also wherever his influence extended. To this end he summoned Guy to Rome and gave him charge of the new hospital of Santo Spirito. Visitors from all parts of the world were shown this hospital and encouraged to establish similar ones in their own communities. The object lesson served such a useful purpose that very soon hospitals were arising in every city of importance in Europe. The "Benificienza Romana" of Querini gives the names of thirty hospitals founded in Rome itself from the eleventh to the fifteenth century.

The part played by the crusades and the military and hospital orders in the evolution of hospitals cannot be overlooked. Disease and pestilence were more potent in defeating the crusaders than the swords of the Saracens, and the military hospital orders found abundant employment. The Knights of St. John, an order founded to care for the sick and wounded, maintained after the conquest a hospital at Jerusalem said to accommodate 2,000 patients. Many priories were established in various parts of Europe while the order flourished. At first the knights acted as nurses and physicians to the sick crusaders; the military features of the order developed later. The organization became very rich and powerful in the course of time, and, swerving from its original purpose, degenerated and finally fell into disrepute. The Teutonic order, an organization of German knights banded together for labor in the Holy Land, did splendid work in building and managing hospitals. Many German hospitals were under its control and, unlike the Knights of St. John, it adhered closely to its original purpose. War and consequent financial reverses caused its dismemberment.

With all these institutions builded by popes, bishops, monks and crusaders, it would seem too soon to look for city hospitals. Yet very many such arose after the first crusade. Eastern commerce flowing in the wake of the crusaders, an increased national wealth and an increased population furnished both the resources for and the need of municipal and privately endowed institutions. Privately endowed hospitals are found first in Italy, and during the twelfth century Monza had three and Milan eleven such institutions. During the fourteenth century Florence had thirty private foundations. Some of the founders were notable people; the Santa Maria Annunziata in Florence was founded by Falco Portinari, father of Dante's Beatrice, and one of the Milan institutions by the Duke Francesco Sforza. In Germany during this period fifty-two city hospitals existed, sixteen being situated in Cologne, the remainder in about thirty smaller cities, the names of which are enumerated by Virchow.

Various abuses began to creep into hospital administration during this period of prosperity which later caused trouble to ecclesiastical authorities, until some of the hospitals, while still conducted by religions orders, were placed under civil authority, the church still paying for their maintenance. In Italy, toward the end of the middle ages, this tendency grew more marked ; in France it came considerably later, although the same conditions existed. It was in the fifteenth century that the Hotel Dieu showed such gross mismanagement that the ecclesiastical chapter of Notre Dame, feeling its inefficiency to cope with the situation, requested the civil authorities to take over the hospital (April, 1505). It was thereafter managed by a board of eight trustees.

The ancient hospitals in Great Britain and France were for a long time under the control of the monastic orders. According to Harduin, a large hospital was founded at St. Albans in a.d. 861. Alcuin, the great scholar, who afterwards was called to the court of Charlemagne to preside over the School of the Palace, wrote to the Archbishop of York (796), and urged the foundation of hospitals for the poor and for pilgrims. The oldest hospital existing to-day as a foundation is St. Bartholomew's in London. This was established in the twelfth century by Rahere, at one time a jester to King Henry I., who later joined a religious community and secured a grant of land near London. Until its disestablishment under Henry VIII. this was the leading London hospital. St. Thomas' hospital, founded in 1215 by Peter, bishop of Winchester, suffered a similar fate, but was reestablished by Edward VI. Among other important hospitals of London belonging to the thirteenth century were Bethlehem, which later became an insane asylum and had its name contracted to Bedlam, Christ's Hospital and the Bridewell, the latter later becoming a prison and the former a school.

There were many other hospitals in England during the middle ages outside of London, and Dugdale in his Monasticum Anglicanum enumerates 460 and gives the charters of many of them.

Prior to the sixteenth century seventy-seven hospitals were founded in Scotland and over twice that number in Ireland. The green island gives testimony as to the existence of hospitals not only by her law- code, the Brehon laws, but also by the perpetuation of such place-names as Spidal, Spital and Hospital. The Brehon laws are specific regarding hospitals, stating that the hospital must be free from debt, must have four doors for ventilation and that a stream of water should run through the middle of the floor. Dogs, fools and scolding women must be kept away from the patient. Whoever injures another must pay for the maintenance of the injured one in the hospital or private house and also for the maintenance of the mother of the injured one, if she should be living. The Knights of St. John established several priories in Ireland, the most important one being Kilmainham priory, founded in 1174 by Strongbow. The Crutched Friars or Crossbearers flourished during the twelfth century and erected many hospitals. There are records of thirteen hospitals founded from this time onward which were confiscated in the strife following the reformation. That a number of leper-houses existed is attested by documentary references as well as by place-names.

Before we pass on to the modern epoch, a consideration of the character and discipline of these medieval hospitals will be of value. With a view probably toward facilitating drainage many of these hospitals were built near a river, as the Hotel Dieu, on the Seine; the Santo Spirito of Borne, on the Tiber ; St. Francis, in Prague ; on the Moldan ; and Mainz, on the Ehine. Many of these early hospitals were small, especially those privately endowed, and contained only about fifteen beds ; others were planned by able architects, and on a large scale. The main ward at Santo Spirito, in Rome, was 409 feet X 40 ; at Tonnere 260 X 60; at Frankford 130 X 40. All these hospitals had numerous windows for ventilation, and some a cupola. The interior was usually decorated with

great skill and care. Says Gardner, in his history
of Siena:

> The hospital at Siena constitutes almost as striking a
> bit of architecture as any edifice of the period and
> contains a magnificent set of frescoes, some of the
> fourteenth century, others later.

The Tonerre hospital, previously referred to,
founded in 1293 by Margaret of Burgundy,
sister-in-law of Louis IX., was situated between
the branches of a small stream, and its ward
was lighted by many large windows extending
high up in the walls. A narrow gallery ran along
the wall twelve feet from the floor for the
regulation of ventilation through the windows
and the seating of convalescent patients in the
sun. The beds were separated by low, wooden
partitions which were portable, making the
alcoved recesses part of one large hall at will,
so that when mass was celebrated in the center

of the building the altar was visible from all parts of the ward.

Mr. Arthur Dillon, an architect, whose scholarly article on this hospital appeared in 1904, says of its construction :

It was an admirable hospital in every way, and it is doubtful if we to-day surpass it. It was isolated, the ward separated from the other buildings, it had the advantage we so often lose of being one story high, and more space was afforded each patient than we can afford.

Now as to the management of these medieval hospitals. In the monasteries the superintendency was in the hands of the abbot or prior and the institution was subject to monastic rule. Even in the privately endowed hospitals practically all the hospital attendants were members of some religious community. How well these communities did their work and with what real humanitarian zeal is attested by Virchow.

In the military orders, the knights called their chief administrative officer commander; in the city hospitals this officer was called magister or rector. The rector was appointed by the bishop, the municipality or the patron. Laymen were eligible for this position and in many legacies lay control was stipulated as a condition. This rector was obliged to take inventories, render and keep accounts, act as trustee for hospital property and frequently to receive and assign patients.

Usually the attendants were males, although in some hospitals male nurses had charge of surgical cases, while females conducted the obstetric and children's wards. Board and clothing were provided these nurses, but no salary. Details of dress, food and recreation were rigidly prescribed, with appropriate penalties for infractions of the rules.

Patients were admitted from all classes and beliefs without qualification, and once admitted the patient was treated as a master of the house, "quasi dominum secundum posse domus," to quote literally from the regulations. He was bathed, his ills attended to, and if a Christian was confessed by the chaplain.

The regulations specified that the sick should never be left unattended, that nurses should be on duty at all hours of the day and night, and that patients dangerously ill should be removed from public wards to a private room. Santo Maria Nuova, at Florence, had a separate ward for delirious patients, and maternity cases were attended in a separate pavilion and kept in the hospital for three weeks after delivery. Sound hygiene is evidenced in numerous regulations concerning changes of bedding, ventilation, and heating by stoves and braziers.

The revenues of the hospitals were derived usually from endowments, either given as private bequests or by church authorities. In times of unusual need special taxes were levied on commodities such as oil, salt, wheat, etc. Some hospitals owned houses, farms, vineyards and even whole villages as sources of income. Various societies and guilds were also established in aid of hospitals, and frequently diocesan laws required the clergy, especially the canons of cathedrals, to contribute. The complete foundations for hospitals, as well as the establishment of beds and contributions for heating and lighting, etc., were frequently made by lay persons.

As the hospitals increased in wealth and the religious orders grew lax in their discipline various abuses arose. Inefficient supervision by ecclesiastical authorities, too many attendants, too few beds, and imposition on the hospital by malingerers were among the evils which ultimately resulted in a loss of efficiency in these institutions. In spite of these drawbacks, however, says Virchow, "we have much to learn from the calumniated middle-ages, much that we with far more abundant means can emulate for the sake of God and man as well."

Pastoral medicine predominated up to the twelfth century and medical as well as surgical treatment was administered by monks and clerics. But with the rise of the university schools of medicine — Salerno, Montpellier, Bologna and Rome — and the development of such surgeons as Wm, Salicetto or Salicet, Henry Mondeville, Lanfranc and Guy de Chauliac during the thirteenth and fourteenth centuries, clerical medical practise began to wane.

It was deemed improper that a priest should shed blood and the church discouraged the practise of surgery by clerics as well as the practise of medicine for fees. Penalties for violating these precepts were laid down at the Council of Clermont (1130), Rheims (1131) and the Second and Fourth Lateran Councils (1134-1215).

The influence of the university-trained physician and surgeon on the hospital dates from this period. More and more we find lay practitioners called to attend hospital patients. In the sixteenth century we find the lay physician's connection with the Italian hospitals to be essentially the same as that in vogue at the present day. In 1524 Henry VIII. received a letter from the rector of the Hospital of Santa Maria Nuova in Florence, answering a request for information concerning the management of that hospital. From this letter we learn that three *adstantes*, or *internes*, attended patients and reported on their condition daily to six visiting physicians from the city. These six visiting physicians then outlined treatment and gave directions for the care of patients. Attached to the hospital was a dispensary for ambulatory cases. This was attended by an eminent surgeon and three assistants, all of whom gave their services without charge. Lallemand in his "*Histoire de la Charité*" gives a list of the many drugs used, and an outline of the pharmacist's duties.

Abuses in management and the civil and religious strife following the Reformation interrupted for a time the progress of the hospital movement. Revenues were cut off and hospital organizations disestablished, especially in England and Germany. It is true that attempts were made to carry on the work by parishes and municipalities, but with indifferent success.

Luther in his letters from Italy shows that he realized the importance of hospital work and he praised the Italian hospitals for their excellence. Meanwhile, a counter-reformation within the church organization was mindful of the hospital. Vives, the humanist of Bruges (1526), made a plea for a census of the inhabitants of cities, the regulation of vagrancy and hospital economy, whereby medical attendance was made more complete and the richer institutions were obliged to share their revenues with the poorer. These salutary reforms were put into practise in Belgium and later were extended by Charles V. to his entire empire. In addition the Council of Trent passed rigid ordinances concerning hospital management and placed hospitals under episcopal supervision in order to prevent abuses and loose practises in administration. With these enactments improvement soon followed, and it is worthy of note that in the hospital at Milan, founded by St. Charles Borromeo, the rules sought to prevent malingering and obliged a strict accounting of its management.

In France the control of hospitals had passed to the king Louis XIV founded a special hospital at Paris for invalids, convalescents and incurables, as well as the great Hospital General for the poor. It was at this time that St. Vincent de Paul began his work and established the Sisters of Charity, a community destined to be famous for its work in camp and battlefield and to exert a tremendous influence on the development of nursing and the building and management of hospitals in all parts of the world. An increasing number of communities of women's nursing orders were formed from the sixteenth century onward until today they practically dominate this field of endeavor.

During the reign of Louis XVI. the Hotel Dieu showed gross mismanagement and a frightful mortality. Sometimes as many as

5,000 patients were crowded there in utter neglect and abandonment. An eminent commission, including in its membership Tenon, Lavoisier and Laplace, was appointed by the king to formulate plans for remedying existing conditions. This board reported in 1788, recommending that certain wards be abandoned and that the pavilion system as exemplified in the hospital at Plymouth, England, be adopted. But the French revolution intervened, and the needed improvements were not made until the nineteenth century.

When we consider the growth in population and wealth of nations and vaunted increase in knowledge, we cannot look upon the eighteenth century as a period fruitful in hospital progress. Many new institutions were erected, it is true, but they were inadequate to the needs of the times in many respects. Among the most important establishments of this period were, in

England: Westminster (1719), Guy's (1722), St. George's (1733); in Germany: the Charite in Berlin, established by Frederick II. (1710), and the Bamburg Hospital, by Bishop Van Erthral (1789) ; in Austria: the famous General Hospital, founded by Joseph II. (1784). Overcrowding, the prevalence of hospital gangrene and erysipelas, and the frightful mortality in many institutions made the very name hospital synonymous in the public mind with suffering and death. Yet, in spite of all this, it is from this very period that we see the development of the idea of the hospital as a necessary adjunct to medical and surgical teaching.

The history of American hospitals begins with the hospital erected by Cortez in the City of Mexico in 1524. It was remembered by the conqueror in his bequests, is still in existence as the Hospital Jesus Nazerino, and the ducal family descended from Cortez, the Dukes of Terranova y Monteleon, still exercise their prerogative of appointing its superintendents. A decade after its establishment came the Hospital of San Lazaro, accommodating 400 patients and, in 1540, the Royal Hospital, both in the City of Mexico.

Bancroft states that the law of 1541 ordered that hospitals be established in all Spanish and Indian towns. The Council of Lima (1583) made provision for the support of hospitals, and two distinct religious orders of men were founded in Mexico for hospital work.

In Canada, the Duchess of Aiguillon founded, in 1639, the Hotel Dieu, at Sillery, afterwards transferred to Quebec. The Hotel Dieu, in Montreal, was founded in 1664; the General Hospital at Quebec in 1693.

The first hospital in the United States territory was erected about 1663 on Manhattan Island to care for ill soldiers and negroes of the East India *Co*. Early in the eighteenth century pest-houses for contagious diseases were established in various towns on the Atlantic coast. A permanent hospital for these ailments was built in Boston in 1717.

One of the petitioners for the incorporation of the Pennsylvania Hospital was Benjamin Franklin. The corner stone was laid in 1755, its charter having been obtained four years previously, but the structure was not completed until 1805.

The first privately endowed hospital established in the United States was the Charity, in New Orleans, founded about 1720 by a sailor named Louis, afterwards an officer in the company of the Indies, who left a small fortune as a foundation. It was destroyed by fire in 1779 and the new Charity Hospital, now the City Hospital, was endowed in 1780. This is now one of the most important hospitals in America and receives over 8,000 patients annually.

The oldest hospital in New York City is the New York Hospital, founded in 1770 by private subscriptions. It was allowed £800 for a period of twenty years by the Municipal Assembly. The state legislature was more generous, allowing it £4,000 annually in 1795 and increasing it in 1796 to £5,000. Bellevue originated in the infirmary attached to the New York City Alms House. It was erected on its present site in 1811. Among the most important sectarian hospitals in New York are St. Vincent's, 1849, St. Luke's, 1850, and Mt. Sinai, 1852.

Fifty-six men of Boston in 1810 addressed a circular letter concerning the establishment in that city of a hospital for the poor. Jackson, Warren, and other medical lights of the day, worked out plans, and the institution, known as the Massachusetts General Hospital, was opened in 1821.

Of existing Baltimore institutions, St. Joseph's was established by the Sisters of St. Joseph in 1864; the Hebrew Hospital in 1867. The Johns Hopkins Hospital, chartered in 1867, was opened in 1889.

The District of Columbia had four hospitals during the cholera epidemic of 1832. The Washington Infirmary received congressional aid and it was proposed to enlarge it into a hospital, but it was burned during the Civil War. The Government Hospital for the Insane was established in 1852 to care for insane cases. Providence Hospital was established in 1861, largely through the efforts of Dr. Toner. Freedman's Hospital was opened in 1862 and Columbia Hospital in 1866. During the war sixty military hospitals were located in Washington and in the vicinity.

In the last half century the spread of hospitals throughout the world received a marvelous impetus. The role of bacteriology as applied to preventive medicine, surgery and therapeutics is one that must be accorded first place in advancing modern hospital efficiency. And in this connection the part played by Virchow's teaching of cellular pathology is a factor of much importance in its influence on medical thought reflected in hospital laboratory methods.

The Franco-Prussian and our own Civil War had much to do with directing men's attention to the problem of hospital construction and military surgery. Improved technique in nursing evolved the modern training school and created a distinctly new profession. Even before Lister's time, Florence Nightingale believed that soap and water and plenty of fresh air and sunlight would lessen mortality from hospital gangrene. Pastor Fleidner, with his training school at Kaiserworth, and the Sisters of Charity in Paris and at the great General Hospital in Vienna, had practised, if they had not preached, this doctrine for a long time. It remained for the Crimean War and the dramatic demonstration of her doctrine by Miss Nightingale to convince the profession at large and the public. How it was accomplished is an oft-told tale. The later teaching of bacteriology in medical schools confirmed the claims for hospital cleanliness; hospital gangrene and epidemic erysipelas have disappeared.

Now is the golden age of the hospital ; we need no statistics to convince us of this. Every American community of any size has not only a hospital, but a training school, and the old public distrust of the institution is on the wane with the improvement in methods and administration. Today the patient approaches it with confidence instead of apprehension, with alacrity instead of with reluctance, and with the hope of life rather than with the fear of death.